The Recipe Makeover Diet

Fight Fat with Healthy Substitutions

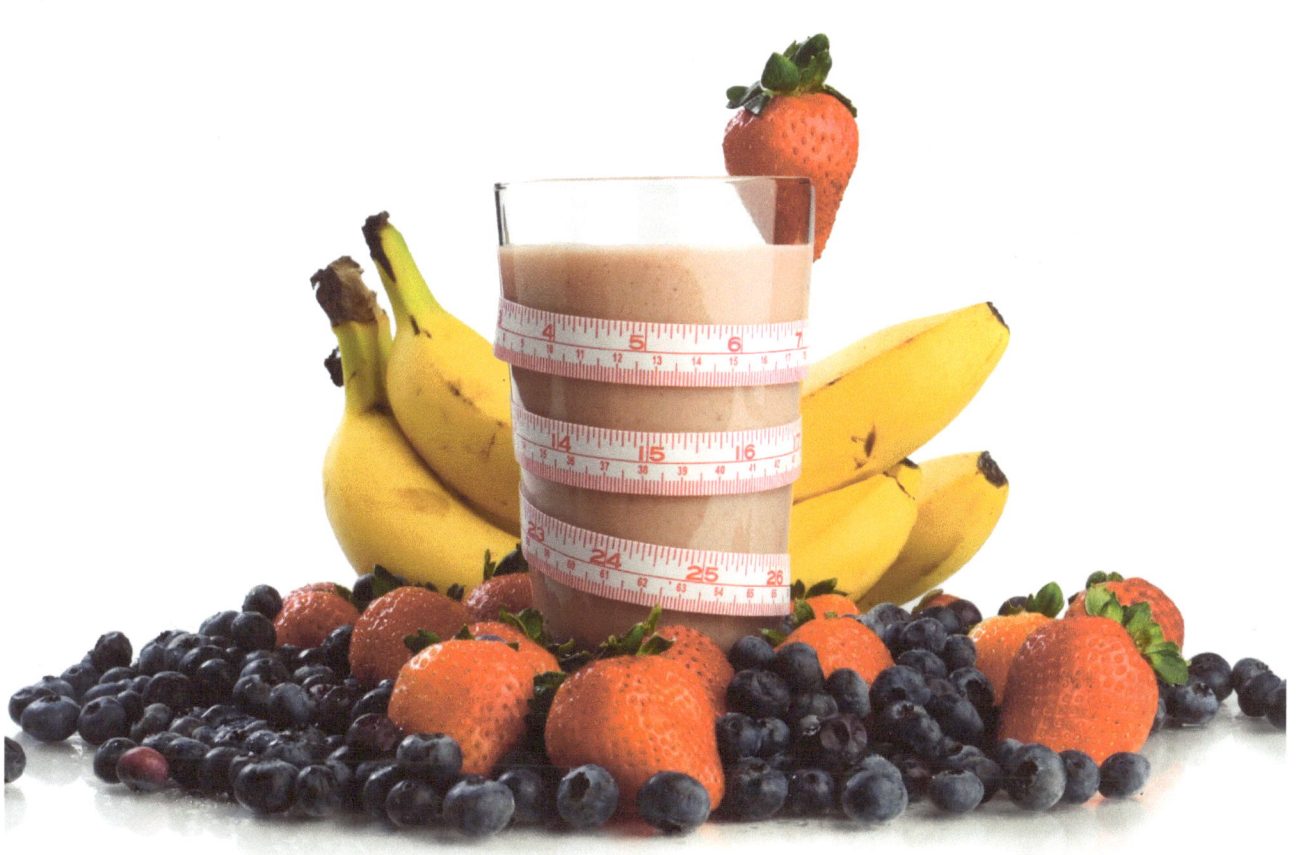

George Rapitis, Dietitian

AuthorHouse™
1663 Liberty Drive
Bloomington, IN 47403
www.authorhouse.com
Phone: 1-800-839-8640

First published by AuthorHouse   6/30/2009

ISBN: 978-1-4389-0786-4 (sc)

Printed in the United States of America
Bloomington, Indiana

This book is printed on acid-free paper.

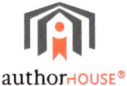

authorHOUSE®

The Recipe Makeover Diet

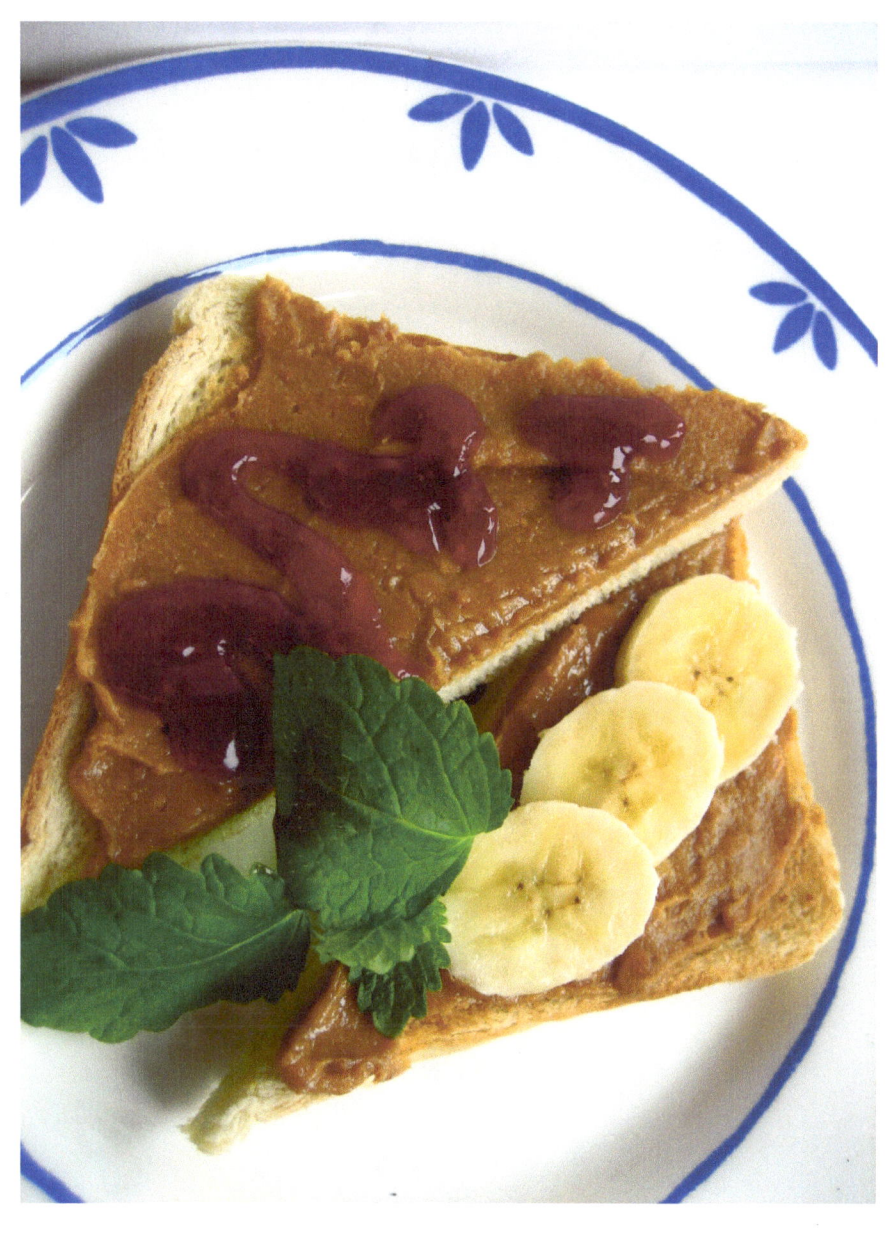

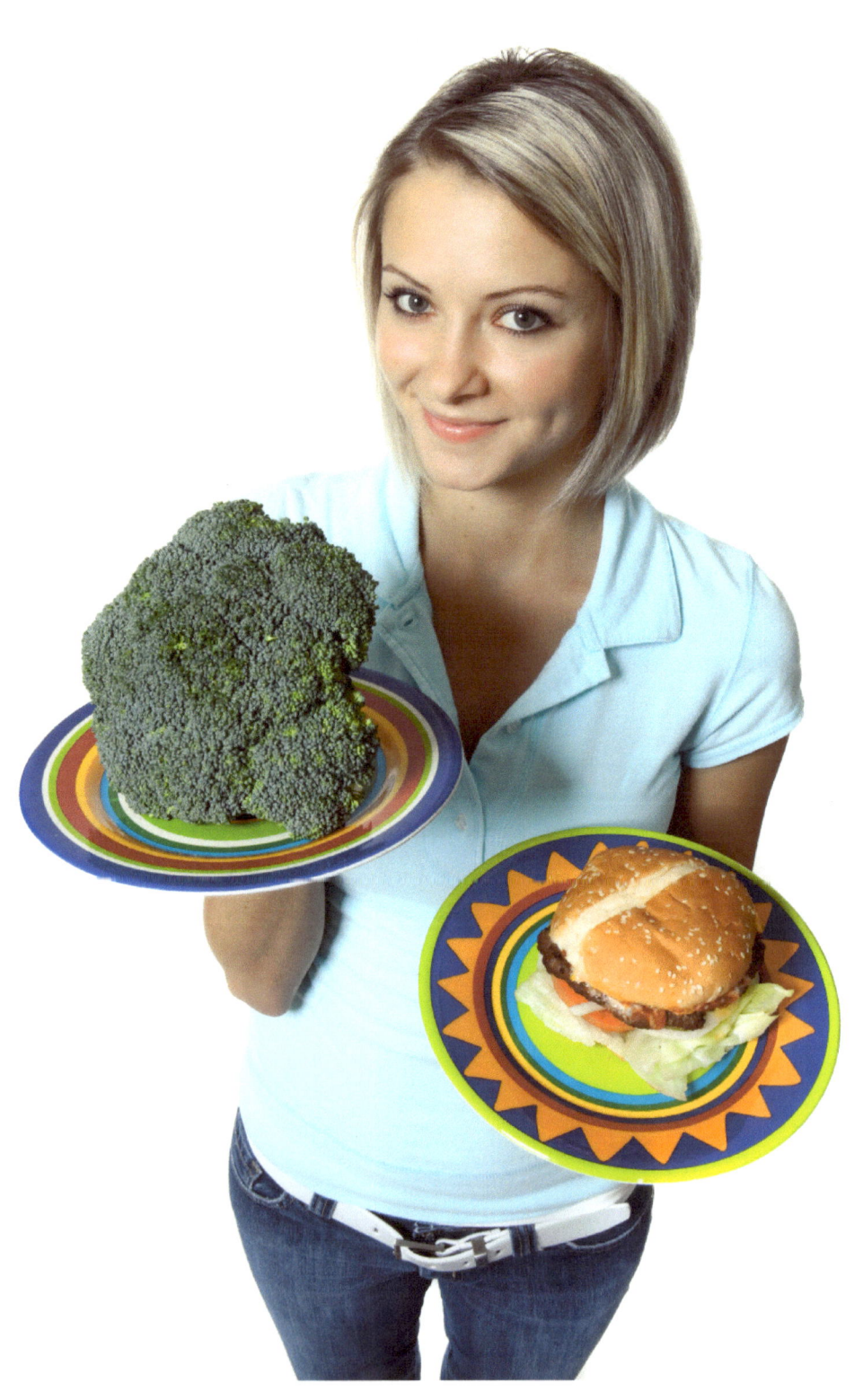

Contents

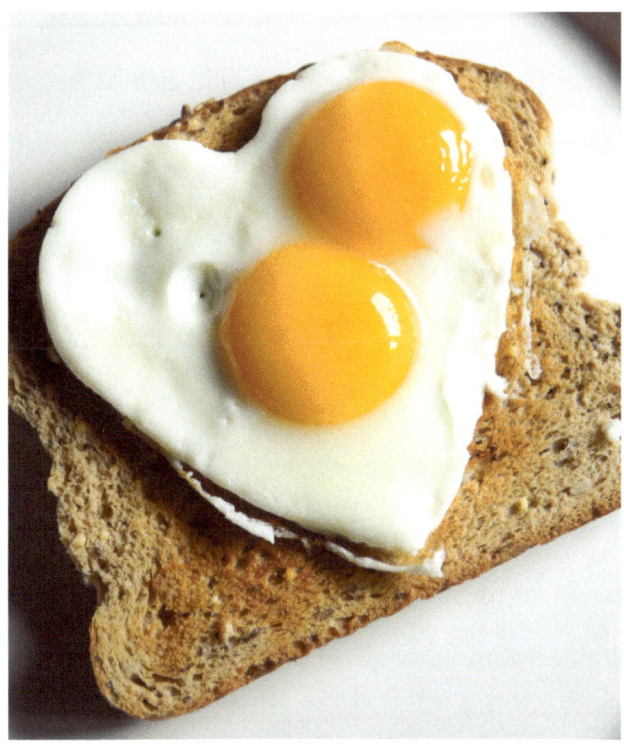

How The Recipe Makeover Diet Works?

The first part of this book contains explains how to cook thin for those wanting to learn healthycooking techniques. The second part contains individual recipemakeovers recipes that show how to cut calories from your diet. The third part of this book contains the the recipemakoverdiet eating plan for 1,500 calories daily. The fourth part contains the diabetes eating guide, gluten free diet and healthy substitution chart.

The *Recipe Makeover Diet* can help you lose up to 10 lbs a month by including the following foods in your diet: nuts, eggs, salmon, low-fat dairy, peanut butter, avocado, spinach, berries, whole grains, and dark chocolate. These fat melting foods burn fat in different ways allowing you to look thinner. The high protein content of nuts and eggs helps curb hunger and boost your calorie burn, meaning you'll eat less (and lose weight). The calcium in dairy trims your waist by increasing the activity of enzymes that break down fat. It also reduces levels of cortisol, a stress hormone that causes your body to hang on to belly flab. Whole grains, leafy greens, and berries are loaded with filling, which has been proven to reduce your calorie intake. The mono- and polyunsaturated fats in peanut butter, avocados, olive oil, and salmon prevent abdominal fat from accumulating in the first place, research shows. And dark chocolate? Indulging in a little bit every day keeps cravings control, which helps you stick to a healthy diet. Get the ab-flattening benefits of these foods with the recipemakeover diet. In addition, this book includes the cooking methods that can make you thinner, recipemakeovers, diabetes eating plan, gluten free sample eating plan, and a healthy cooking subsitution eating chart. Important Disclaimer: This book is not a replacement for medical advice. Users should consulta health professional before making any health decisions based on material contained herein.

Introduction - Portion Distortion

As the portion size of the average American meal grows, so have Americans waistlines. In fact, according to the Centers for Disease Control, the numbers of Americans who are considered obese by body mass index (or have a BMI score of 30 or greater), and the number of obese keeps rising every year. In addition, food portions are 2 to 5 times larger then they have ever been as a result of people not using moderation when making food choices. The answer to the obesity and portion distortion epidemic is making healthy changes in our eating habits by choosing fat fighting foods. By following the recipes in this eating plan, you will no longer need large portion sizes. In this eating plan you will eat three meals and two snacks a day each with a healthy dose of the fat fighting foods. You can repeat meals to maximize your food dollars or to replace one you don't care for. For free access to more meals to follow, visit www.planetyorgos. com   Ready to start losing weight?

Portion Distortion

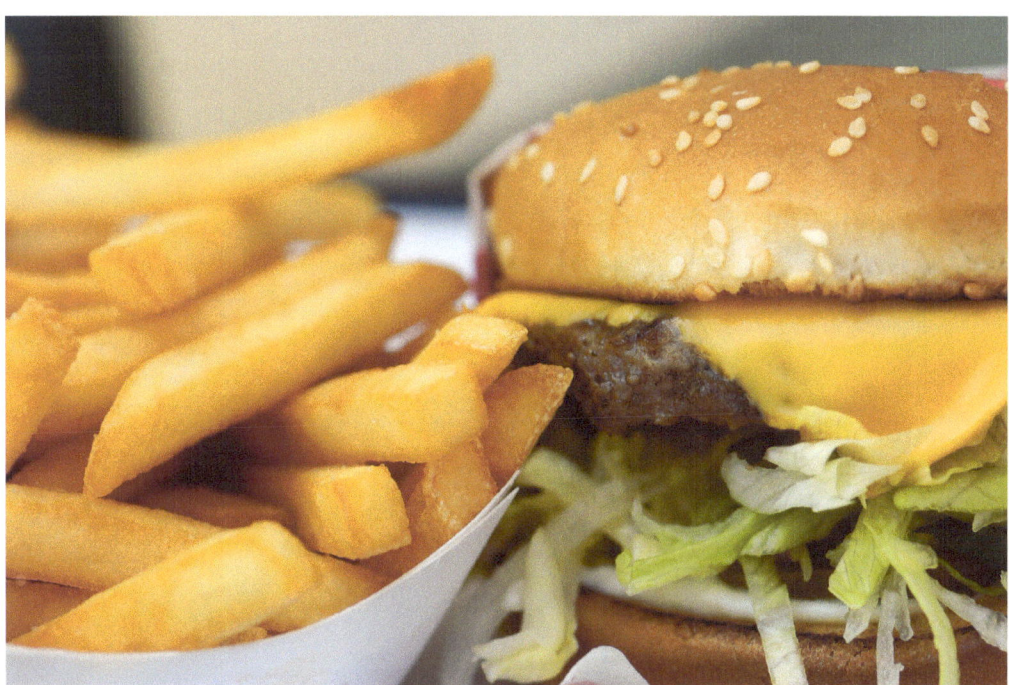

Roasted Lamb Chops

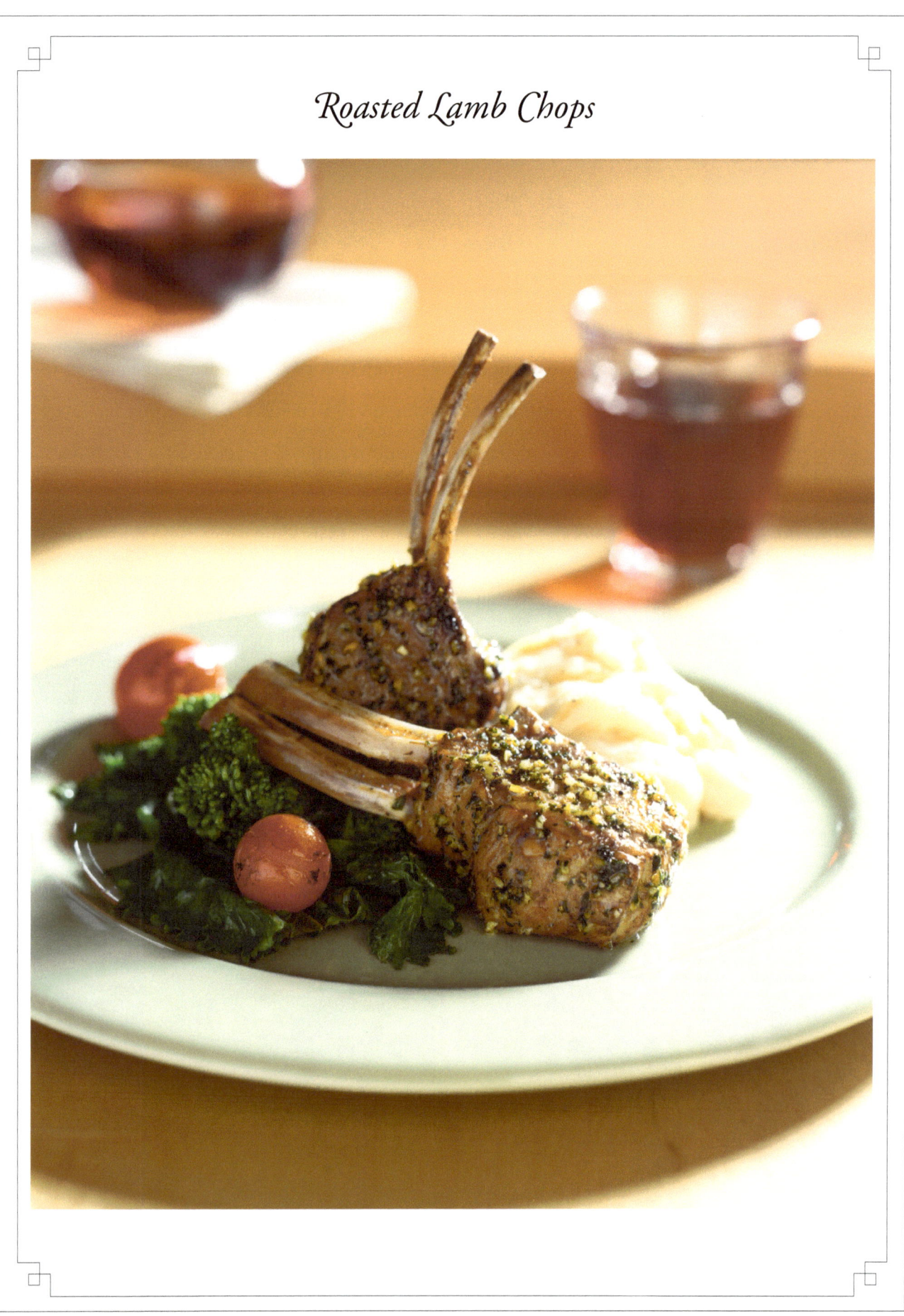

Chapter 1 - Thin Cooking Methods

A healthful eating plan means more than choosing the right foods to eat. Some ways of cooking are better than others when it comes to cutting cholesterol, fat and calories. You don't have to give up taste for the things you enjoy eating. Just learn some healthful cooking techniques and you can have it all (almost)!

What are thin cooking methods?

- *Roast-* with a rack so the meat or poultry doesn't sit in its own fat drippings. Set at 350 degrees to avoid searing. Baste with fat free liquids such as wine, tomato juice or lemon juice.

- *Bake-* in covered cookware with a little extra liquid.

- *Braise or stew-* with more liquid than baking, on top of the stove or in the oven. Refrigerate the cooked dish and remove the chilled fat before reheating.

- *Poach-* by immersing chicken or fish in the simmering liquid.

- *Grill or broil-* on a rack so fat drips away from the food.

- *Sauté-* in an open skillet over high heat. Use nonstick vegetable spray, a small amount of broth or wine or a tiny bit of canola oil rubbed onto the pan with a paper towel.

- *Steam-* in a basket over simmering water.

How can you cut fat without losing taste?

- After browning, ground meat should be put into a strainer lined with paper towels.

- When making gravy without fat, blend a tablespoon of cornstarch with a cup of broth by shaking them together in a jar. Heat rest of the broth and add the blended liquid, simmering until thick.

- When preparing scrambled eggs or omelets use only one egg yolk per portion, and add a few extra egg whites to the batch. Or use an egg substitute product.

- Remove oils by draining canned tuna, salmon or sardines and rinsing them in water.

- Vegetables should not be overcooked. Steaming or baking them instead of boiling so they keep more of their natural flavors.

- Using finely chopped vegetables to stretch ground poultry or meat.

- Using herbs and spices to add flavor to foods.

Chapter 2 - The Meal Makeover

The biggest strides in cutting saturated fat come from halving average red meat portions and switching from full fat dairy to the reduced fat variety. Trimming saturated fat allows you to double up on fruits and vegetables. In addition you will double up on food overall helping you feel more full and satisfied.

Average American Meal

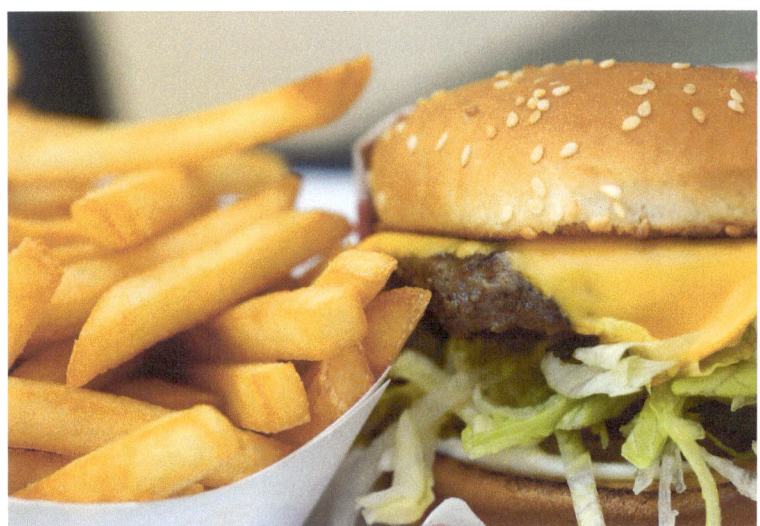

Eating fattier cuts of meat in larger serving sizes such as in the average American meal allows fat and calories to add up.

Remodeled Meal

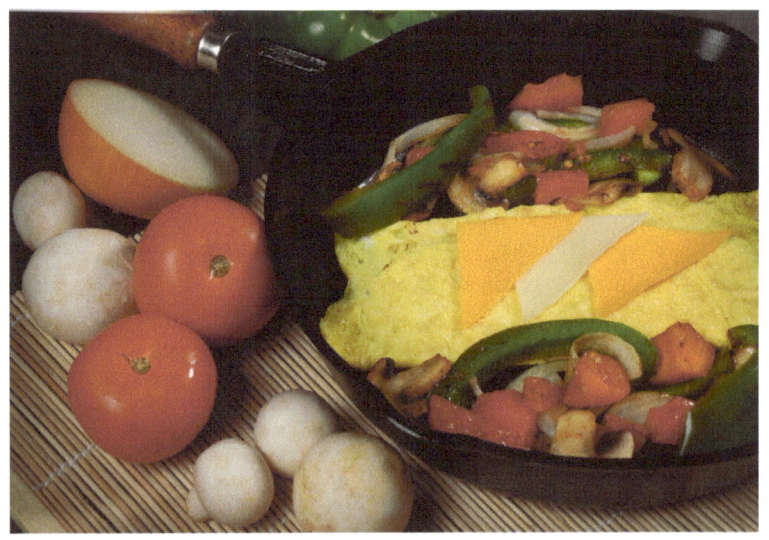

Incorporate meat into a vegetable-laden omelet, keeping the portion size smart. Serve with a variety of vegetables.

Chapter 3 - Recipe Makeovers

Healthy substitutions not only reduce the amount of fat, calories and sodium in your recipes, but also can boost the nutritional content. For example, use whole-wheat pasta in place of enriched pasta. You'll triple the fiber and reduce the number of calories. Prepare a dessert with fat-free milk instead of whole milk to save 63 calories and almost 8 grams of fat per cup. In some recipes, you can delete an ingredient altogether; likely candidates include items such as frostings which are high in fat and calories. Other possibilities include optional condiments, butter, mayonnaise, which can have large amounts of fat and calories. Try green tea instead of sodas.

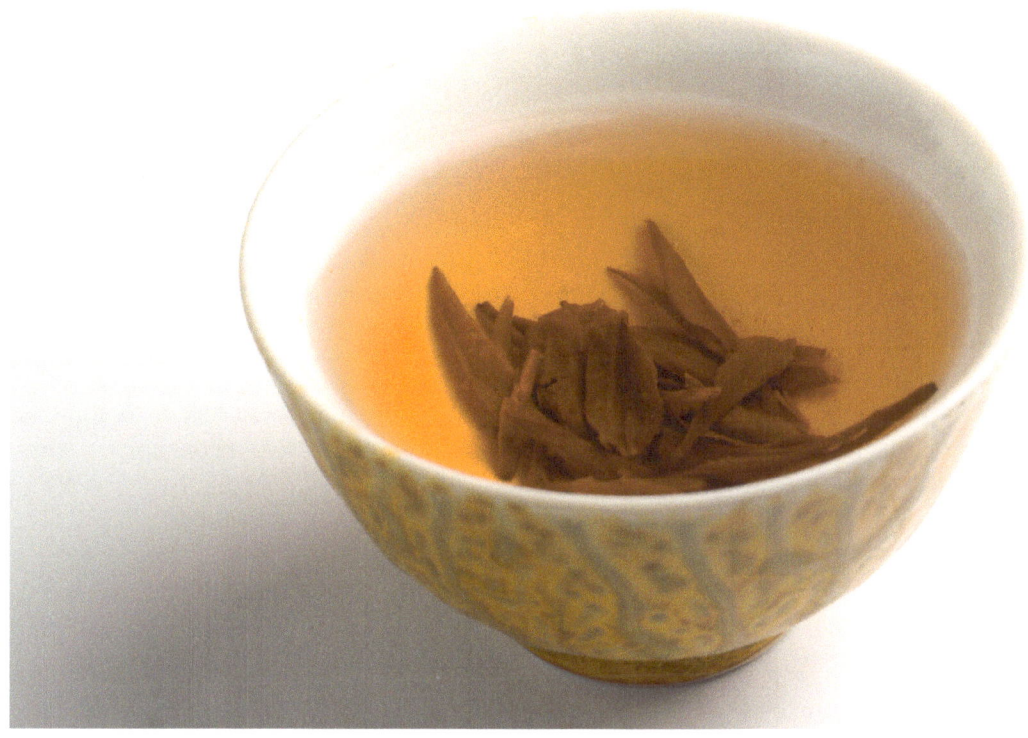

Many recipes can tolerate a healthy renovation without affecting the taste or texture of the food. So whether trying to stick to a healthy-eating plan or following a special diet, these techniques to make recipes delicious and nutritious.

Apple Stuffed Tenderloin with Cinnamon Raisin Sauce

This hearty entrée started out as stuffed pork chops. But, to make the dish leaner and still keep its character, switch to pork tenderloin. Calories, fat and cholesterol were reduced by:

Using pork tenderloin (26% calories from fat) instead of rib chops (52 % calories from fat), using non-stick spray instead of butter to sauté the onions and eliminating the butter in the sauce.

Stuffed Pork Tenderloin

- 1 pork tenderloin (1-1 ½ lbs) trimmed of all visible fat
- 2 med. oranges
- 1 med. Apple, cored and chopped
- 2 T. finely chopped onions
- 2/3 cup fine dry plain bread crumbs

Sauce

- 1 c. unsweetened apple juice
- 1 T. cornstarch
- ¼ tsp. Ground cinnamon
- ¼ c. raisins

Directions: Preheat oven to 425 degrees. Cut a pocket in the side of the tenderloin by cutting a lengthwise slit from one side to almost the other side and stopping ½ inch from each of the tapered ends. Set the tenderloin aside. Finely shred the peel from the oranges and set aside. Squeeze juice from oranges. In a medium bowl, combine the orange juice and apples and set aside. Spray an unheated small skillet with non-stick spray. Add onions. Cook and stir over medium heat until tender. Then add the onions and breadcrumbs to the apple mixture. Toss until combined. Spoon the bread mixture into the pocket of the tenderloin. Securely close the pocket with wooden toothpicks. Place the tenderloin on a rack in a shallow roasting pan. Insert a meat thermometer into the meat portion only. Bake for 25 to 30 minutes or until the thermometer registers 160 degrees. Let stand about 5 min. before slicing.

To make sauce: In a small saucepan, use a wire whisk to stir together 2 tablespoons of the apple juice and the cornstarch. Then stir in remaining apple juice. Cook and stir over medium heat until boiling. Stir in the reserved orange peel and cinnamon. Add the raisins and cook for 5 minutes, stilling occasionally. To serve, slice the tenderloin. Spoon the sauce over the slices.

Makes 4 servings.

Meatless Moussaka

Here's a new twist on a traditional Greek Favorite. It's much leaner then a standard recipe, which could easily cost you 40 grams of fat per serving. Replacing the rich cream sauce with a fresh tomato sauce made with the biggest difference. This recipe was made over by:

Replacing the lamb with tofu, eliminating the butter, eggs, flour, and milk, eliminating the feta cheese, and reducing the amount of parmesan cheese

- 1 large red onion, thinly sliced and separated into rings
- 1 med. Eggplant, cut crosswise into ½ inch thick rounds
- 2 med. Zucchini, thinly sliced
- 8 oz. firm tofu, crumbled
- ¼ c. minced fresh basil
- 2 T. minced fresh parsley
- 3 c. low- sodium tomato sauce
- ½ t. Frank's hot sauce
- 2 T. grated Parmesan cheese

Directions: Layer the onions, eggplant and zucchini in the bottom of an 11x7 inch-baking dish. Sprinkle the tofu over the vegetables. Then top with basil and parsley. Stir together the tomato sauce and Frank's hot sauce. Pour over the tofu and vegetables. Bake at 350 degrees for 30-40 minutes or until bubbly and the vegetables are tender. Sprinkle with the cheese before serving.

Makes 4 servings.

Hawaiian Chicken

Here's a recipe for classic sweet and sour chicken that's healthier and less messy than usual. Instead of dipping the chicken into a thin batter and deep-frying it, dust the chicken with flour, pan-fry until golden and then finish it off in the oven. Doing the following reduced calories, fat and cholesterol:

Using chicken breasts without the skin, using pineapple canned in its own juice, reducing the amount of sugar, and using non-stick cooking spray instead of oil.

Chicken

- 4 (4 oz.) skinless, boneless chicken breasts
- 1 4-cup whole-wheat flour

Sauce

- 1 (20 oz.) can unsweetened pineapple juice
- ¾ c. sugar
- ½ c. cider vinegar
- 2 T. cornstarch
- 1 tsp. Grated ginger root
- 1 t. chicken broth
- 1 large green pepper, cut into ¼ inch thick rings
- Hot cooked brown rice (optional)

Directions: Preheat oven to 375 degrees. Spray a large skillet with non-stock spray. Heat. Meanwhile, coat both sides of the chicken with the flour. Add chicken to the skillet and brown on both sides. Transfer the chicken to an 8 x 8 – 2-inch baking dish; set aside.

Drain the pineapple, reserving the juice. Transfer the juice to a 2-cup measuring cup. Add enough water to make 1 ¼ cups. In a med. Saucepan, use a wire whisk to stir together the juice mixture, sugar, vinegar, cornstarch, ginger, and broth. Bring to a boil over medium heat. Slightly reduce the heat and gently boil for 4 min., stirring often. Pour half of the sauce over the chicken. Arrange the pineapple slices and pepper rings on top. Then pour on the remaining sauce mixture. Bake for 30 to 40 minutes or until the chicken is tender and no longer pink. Serve with the brown rice.

Sunshine Halibut

When serving fresh halibut, make sure its delicate flavor shins through. In this recipe, you can do that by using only freshly squeezed orange and lemon juices. Calories, fat and cholesterol were reduced by:

Using non-stick cooking spray instead of butter to sauté the vegetables.

Ingredients

- 4 (4 oz.) fresh halibut steaks, cut ¾ inch thick
- 1/3 cup finely chopped onions
- 1 clove garlic, minced
- 2 T. fresh parsley
- ½ t. finely shredded orange peel
- 1/8 t. ground black pepper
- ¼ c. fresh orange juice
- 1 T. fresh lemon juice

Directions: Preheat oven to 400 degrees. Arrange an 8 x 8 – 2-inch baking dish; set aside. Lightly spray an unheated small skillet with no-stick spray. Add the onions and garlic. Cook and stir over medium heat until the onions are tender. Remove the skillet from the heat. Stir in the parsley, orange peel and pepper. Spread the onion mixture on top of the fish. In a custard cup, stir together the orange and lemon juices. Then pour the juice mixture over the fish. Cover with foil and bake for 10-15 minutes or until the fish flakes easily when tested with a fork.

Makes 4 servings.

Poached Salmon with Greek Cucumber Sauce

Here's a classic salmon recipe with a Greek twist. It is important to eat more salmon and here's an easy and delicious way to do it. This recipe is made healthier because the salmon is poached instead of fried and also because:

Omega-3 fats in salmon relieve the inflammation caused by intense workouts.
Yogurt is packed with active cultures that lower your chances of gum disease.
Mint provides menthol with helps quell indigestion.
Orzo provides a hefty dose of long lasting energy.

- 1 (2 lb) Salmon filet with skin
- 2 cups dry white wine
- 2 c. water
- 2 bay leaves
- 2 sprigs flat-leaf parsley
- 2 lemons, unpeeled, sliced
- 1 scallion, top only, thinly sliced
- 1 cup Greek Cucumber sauce (recipe below)

Sauce

- 1 Cucumber
- 1 c. plain, nonfat yogurt drained
- ½ t. minced garlic
- 1 tsp. Olive oil
- 1 t. chopped mint
- 2 tsp. Lemon juice
- ¼ tsp. Lemon zest

Directions: Place wine, water, bay leaves, parsley, and 1 sliced lemon into a large skillet; bring to a simmer. Add salmon, skin side down. Cover skillet and simmer over low heat until the fish is just cooked through about 8 minutes. Transfer fish to a plate, cover, and refrigerate until completely chilled about 3 hours. Peel skin from fillet and scrape away any brown flesh. Serve fish over sautéed baby spinach and top with the scallion, remaining lemon slices, and Greek cucumber sauce. Serve over a cup of cooked orzo.

Chicken Souvlaki with Greek Cucumber Sauce

This healthy traditional Greek recipe only takes 30 minutes prepare including marinating time. Here is the nutritional breakdown:

Calories 140
Fat . . . . 5 g
Cholesterol . . . . .161 mg
Fiber . . . . .2 g
Carbohydrates . . . . . . .31 g

Ingredients

Souvlaki

- 3 T. fresh lemon juice
- 1 ½ t. chopped fresh oregano or ½ dried
- 2 t. olive oil
- ½ t. salt
- 4 garlic cloves, minced
- ½ pound skinless, boneless chicken cut into 1 inch pieces
- 1 med. Zucchini, cut into ½ inch thick slices.
- Nonstick cooking spray.

Greek Cucumber sauce:

- ½ c. cucumber, peeled, seeded and shredded.
- ½ c. plain low-fat yogurt
- 1 T. lemon juice
- ¼ t. salt
- 1 clove garlic, peeled, minced

Serves 2

Directions: To prepare souvlaki, in a plastic sealable bag combine the lemon juice, oregano, olive oil, salt and garlic. Seal bag and shake to combine. Add the chicken to bag; seal and shake to coat. Marinate chicken in refrigerator for 30 minutes, turning once.Remove chicken from bag, discard marinade. Thread the chicken and zucchini alternately onto each of 4 (8 inch) skewers. Coat a grill pan with cooking spray and heat over medium-high heat. Add skewers; cook 8 minutes or until chicken is done, turning once. To prepare sauce, stir together all the sauce ingredients. Serve sauce with souvlaki.

Chocolate Chip-Oatmeal Cookies

Revamped, these gems are still ooey-gooey good — but they're only 80 calories each (with a gram of healthy fiber per cookie). We've also cut out half the fat and cholesterol. Lose the guilt — and indulge!

Ingredients

- 1/2 cup(s) (packed) brown sugar
- 1/2 cup(s) granulated sugar
- 1/2 cup(s) trans fat–free vegetable oil spread (60% to 70% oil)
- 1 large egg
- 1 large egg white
- 2 teaspoon(s) vanilla extract
- 1 1/4 cup(s) all-purpose flour
- 1 teaspoon(s) baking soda
- 1/2 teaspoon(s) salt
- 2 1/2 cup(s) quick-cooking or old-fashioned oats, uncooked
- 1 cup(s) bittersweet (62% cacao) or semisweet chocolate chips

Directions: Preheat oven to 350 degrees F. In large bowl, with mixer on medium-low speed, beat sugars and vegetable spread until well blended, occasionally scraping bowl with rubber spatula. Add egg, egg white, and vanilla; beat until smooth. Beat in flour, baking soda, and salt until mixed. With wooden spoon, stir in oats and chocolate chips until well combined. Drop dough by rounded measuring tablespoons, 2 inches apart, on ungreased large cookie sheet. Bake cookies 12 to 13 minutes or until golden. With wide metal spatula, transfer cookies to wire rack to cool. Repeat until all batter is used. Store cooled cookies in tightly sealed containers up to 3 days.

Nutritional Information: Calories 80, Total fat 4g, Carbohydrates 11g, Fiber 1g, Cholesterol 4mg
(per serving)

Healthy Brownies

The rich texture and chocolatey goodness of these bake-sale favorites speak of decadence, but compare each square's 95 calories, 3 grams of fat, and 0 cholesterol to a regular brownie's doubly high calories, nearly quadrupled fat, and 60 milligrams of cholesterol, and you'll feel virtuous (and satisfied). Our cheats? Swapping nonfat cocoa for chocolate and cholesterol-free spread for not-so-heart-healthy butter.

Ingredients

- 1 teaspoon(s) instant coffee powder or granules
- 2 teaspoon(s) vanilla extract
- 1/2 cup(s) all-purpose flour
- 1/2 cup(s) unsweetened cocoa
- 1/4 teaspoon(s) baking powder
- 1/4 teaspoon(s) salt
- 1 cup(s) sugar
- 1/4 cup(s) trans-fat free vegetable oil spread
- 3 large egg whites

Directions: Preheat oven to 350°F. Grease 8" by 8" metal baking pan. In cup, dissolve coffee in vanilla extract. On waxed paper, combine flour, cocoa, baking powder, and salt. In medium bowl, whisk sugar, vegetable oil spread, egg whites, and coffee mixture until well mixed; then blend in flour mixture. Spread in prepared pan. Bake 22 to 24 minutes or until toothpick inserted in brownies 2 inches from edge comes out almost clean. Cool in pan on wire rack, about 2 hours. When cool, cut brownies into 4 strips, then cut each strip crosswise into 4 squares. If brownies are difficult to cut, dip knife in hot water; wipe dry, and cut. Repeat dipping and drying as necessary.

Nutrition information: Calories 95, Total fat 3g, Carbohydrates 17g, Fiber 1g, Cholesterol 0 mg
(per serving)

Fat Burning Meals

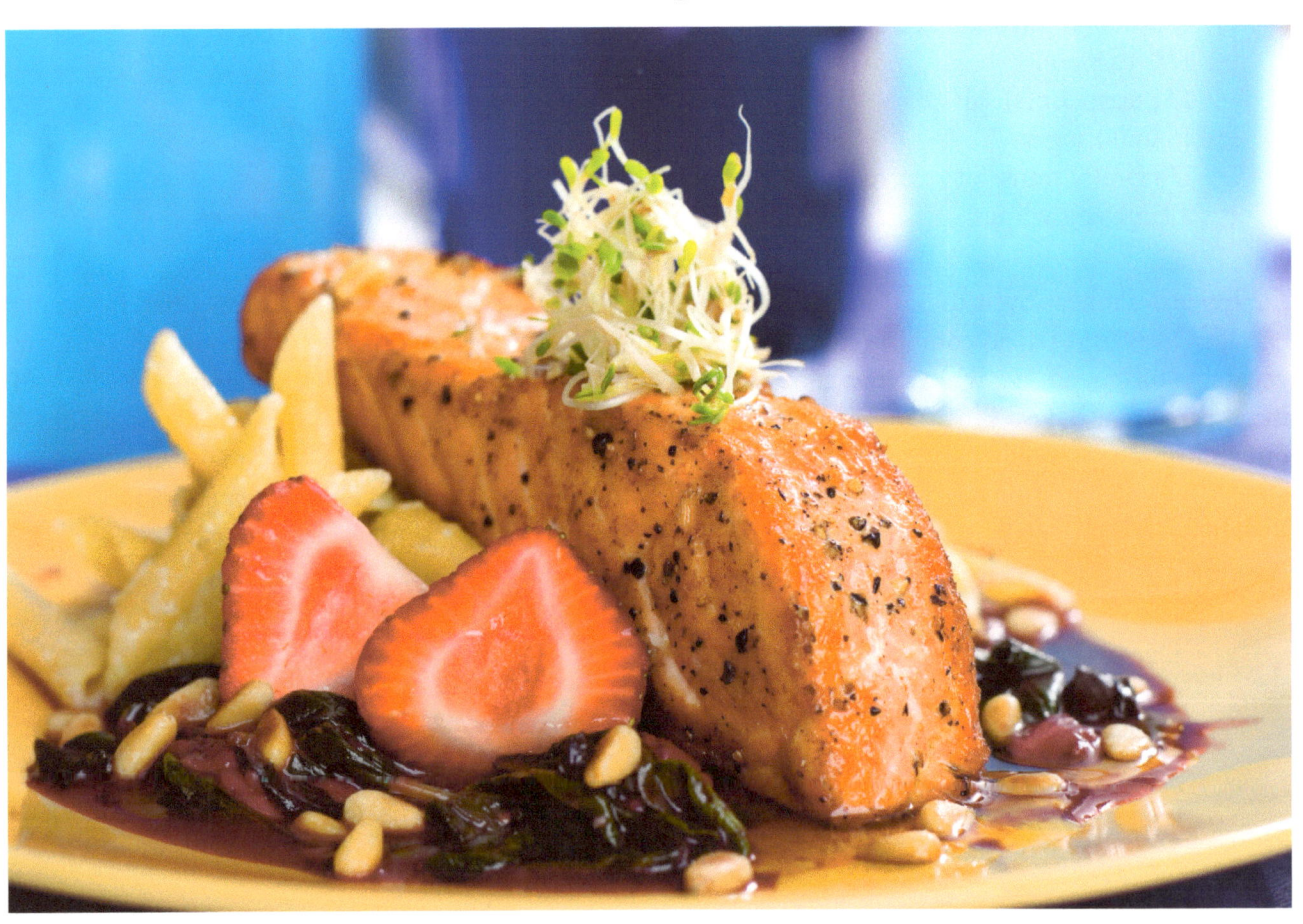

Chapter 4 - Daily Fat Burning Meals

Recipes on the following pages, total 1,500 calories a day. They can help a person lose 8-10 lbs monthly. The fat fighting menu includes: nuts, eggs, salmon, low-fat dairy, peanut butter, avocado, spinach, berries, whole grains, and dark chocolate. Each of these foods works in a different way to fat and make a person sleeker.

The high protein content of nuts and eggs helps curb hunger and boost your calorie burn, meaning you'll eat less (and lose weight). The calcium in dairy products trims your waist by increasing the activity of enzymes that break down fat cells. It also reduces levels of cortisol, a stress hormone that causes your body to hang on to belly flab, Whole grains, leafy greens, and berries are loaded with filling fiber, which has been proven to reduce your calorie intake. The mono- and polyunsaturated fats in peanut butter, avocados, olive oil, and salmon prevent abdominal fat from accumulating in the first place, research shows. And dark chocolate indulging in a little bit every day keeps cravings under control, which helps you stick to a healthy diet.

The ab-flattening benefits of these foods can be used with the following recipes:

Weekly Fat Burning Breakfast Recipes

Chocolate and Peanut Butter Surprise Smoothie

In a blender, combine 3/4 cup frozen berries, 1/4 cup low-fat vanilla yogurt, 1/2 cup low-fat chocolate soy milk, and 2 tablespoons reduced-fat all-natural peanut butter. **355 calories**

Egg-White Mouthwatering Muffin Melt

Scramble 3 egg whites. Cover half of a whole-grain English muffin with 1/2 cup spinach and the other half with 1 slice reduced-fat cheddar cheese; toast until cheese is melted. Add egg and 1 slice tomato. **270 calories**

Berry Good Parfait

Top 1/2 cup low-fat Greek yogurt with 1/4 cup low-fat granola, 1 teaspoon slivered almonds, 1 tablespoon honey, and 1/2 cup berries. **303 calories**

Cinnamon-Apple Oats

Prepare 1 packet plain, instant oatmeal with 1/2 cup skim milk. Microwave 3/4 of a small apple, chopped, 1 teaspoon cinnamon, and 1 teaspoon brown sugar. Top oatmeal with apples and 1 tablespoon chopped walnuts. **255 calories**

Mexican Egg Scramble

Scramble 3 egg whites with 1/4 cup canned black beans (rinsed and drained) and 1 ounce reduced-fat cheddar cheese. Top with 2 tablespoons salsa, or to taste. **191 calories**

Peanut Buttery Bagel

Toast a whole-grain bagel and spread with 1 tablespoon reduced-fat all-natural peanut butter. Cover with slices from 1 apple. **335 calories**

Berry Waffles

Top 2 whole-grain waffles with 1/4 cup low-fat plain yogurt, 1/2 cup mixed berries, and 2 teaspoons maple syrup. **246 calories**

Weekly Fat Burning Lunch Recipes

Turkey-Avocado Melt

Place 2 to 3 slices roasted turkey, 2 slices avocado, and 1 slice low-fat pepper jack cheese between 2 slices whole-grain bread. Grill in skillet. **303 calories**

Penne with Feta and Sun-Dried Tomatoes

Toss 1/2 cup cooked whole wheat pasta with 1 cup sauteed spinach and 2 tablespoons each pine nuts and low-fat feta. Sprinkle with capers and chopped sun-dried tomatoes. **378 calories**

Guacamole Burger

Cook a veggie burger according to package directions. Mash half an avocado with 1/2 cup salsa. Top burger with avocado mixture; serve on a whole-grain bun. **396 calories**

Udon-Tofu Soup

Combine 1/2 cup cooked udon with 1 cup spinach and 1 1/2 cups hot vegetable broth. Add 1/2 cup cubed tofu, 1/2 cup chopped mushrooms, and 1 teaspoon soy sauce. **226 calories**

Spinach Flatbread Pizza

Spread 1/3 cup tomato sauce on 1 naan. Top with 2 cups spinach, 1/4 cup low-fat mozzarella cheese, and 1 tablespoon slivered almonds. Bake at 350 degrees F. until melted. **366 calories**

Zesty Black Beans

Cook 1/2 cup each black beans, chopped bell pepper, and chopped onion and 1 chopped jalapeno in a pan with 2 teaspoons olive oil for 5 minutes. Place over cooked brown rice; top with 1/4 avocado, sliced. **305 calories**

Chopped Chicken Salad

Place 3 ounces chopped chicken, 2 tablespoons crumbled low-fat blue cheese, 1/2 cup chopped cucumber, and 1 tablespoon each chopped pecans and dried cranberries on 2 cups lettuce. Toss with 2 tablespoons vinaigrette. **356 calories**

Weekly Fat Burning Dinner Recipes

Maple Salmon with Greens, Edamame, and Walnuts

Makes: 4 servings

Ingredients

- 3 tablespoons pure maple syrup
- 2 tablespoons balsamic vinegar
- 1 tablespoon lemon juice
- 1 tablespoon Dijon mustard
- 1 tablespoon finely chopped shallot
- 1/4 teaspoon salt
- 1/4 teaspoon freshly ground black pepper
- 2 tablespoons olive oil
- 2 teaspoons snipped fresh rosemary
- 4 5-ounce fresh or frozen skinless salmon fillets, about 1 inch thick
- 1 6-ounce package fresh baby spinach
- 1/2 cup cooked shelled edamame
- 1/2 cup red bell pepper strips
- 1/4 cup chopped walnuts, toasted

Directions: 1. In a small saucepan, combine maple syrup, vinegar, lemon juice, mustard, shallot, salt, and pepper. For dressing, in a small bowl, stir together 2 tblespoons of the maple syrup mixture and the olive oil; set aside. 2. For glaze, heat the remaining maple syrup mixture to boiling; reduce heat. Simmer, uncovered, about 5 minutes, or until syrupy. Remove from heat; stir in rosemary. 3. Preheat broiler. Place fish on the greased, unheated rack of a broiler pan and brush with half the glaze. Broil 6 to 7 inches from heat for 5 minutes. Turn fish over; brush with remaining glaze. Broil for 3 to 5 minutes more, or until fish begins to flake when tested with a fork. 4. Meanwhile, in a large bowl, combine spinach, edamame, pepper strips, and nuts. Drizzle spinach mixture with dressing; toss to coat. Spoon salad onto plates; top with fish.

Nutrition facts per serving: 460 calories, 33g protein, 18g carbohydrate, 28 g fat (5g saturated), 3g fiber

Baked Veggie Omelet

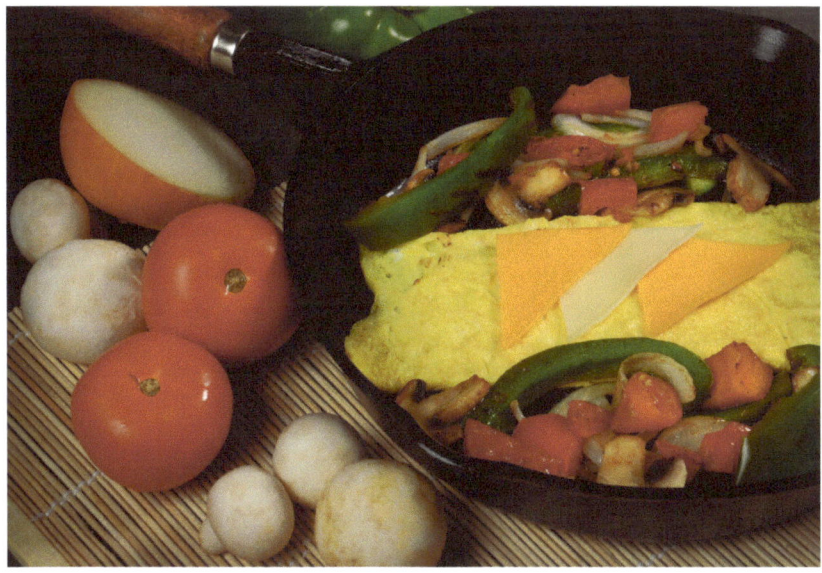

Makes: 6 servings

Ingredients

- Nonstick cooking spray
- 2 tablespoons butter
- 3 cups bite-size bell pepper strips, sliced mushrooms, and thinly sliced zucchini
- 1/3 cup chopped onion (1 small)
- 1/2 teaspoon dried basil
- 1/8 teaspoon black pepper
- 1/2 teaspoon salt
- 3 tablespoons tomato sauce
- 10 egg whites
- 5 eggs
- 1/4 cup water
- 1/4 cup shredded mozzarella cheese
- 2 tablespoons grated Parmesan cheese
- Tomato sauce, warmed (optional)

Directions: 1. Preheat oven to 400 degrees F. Lightly coat a 15-x-10-x-1-inch baking pan with cooking spray; set aside.2. In a large skillet, melt butter over medium heat. Add vegetables, onion, and dried basil. Cook and stir 5 to 8 minutes. Add pepper and 1/4 teaspoon of the salt. Remove from heat; stir in tomato sauce; keep warm.3. In a medium bowl beat egg whites, eggs, water, and remaining 1/4 teaspoon salt with a whisk until combined but not frothy. Pour eggs into the baking pan. Bake uncovered, 7 minutes, or until eggs have just set. 4. Meanwhile, in a small bowl, combine cheeses; set aside.5. Cut the baked eggs into six 5-inch squares. Using a spatula, lift each square fromthe pan and invert onto a plate. Divide warm vegetable mixture among omelets; top with cheese. Fold omelets diagonally in half, forming triangles. If desired, drizzlewith additional tomato sauce.

Nutrition facts per serving: 170 calories, 14g protein, 7g carbohydrate, 10g fat (4g saturated), 2g fiber

Strawberry Chicken Salad with Warm Citrus Dressing

Makes: 4 servings

Ingredients

- 4 medium skinless, boneless chicken-breast halves (about 1 pound)
- 1 14-1/2-ounce can chicken broth
- 2 1/2 cups strawberries
- 1/3 cup orange juice
- 2 tablespoons salad oil
- 2 teaspoons finely shredded lemon peel
- 1 tablespoon lemon juice
- 1 teaspoon sugar
- 1/2 teaspoon chili powder
- 1/4 teaspoon salt
- 1/4 teaspoon freshly ground black pepper
- 6 cups torn spinach, watercress and/or other greens
- 1/4 cup chopped walnuts, toasted

Directions: 1. Sprinkle the chicken-breast halves lightly with salt and pepper. Pour chicken broth into a large saucepan; add chicken. Bring broth to a boil; reduce heat. Cover and simmer for 15 to 20 minutes, or until chicken is tender and no longer pink. Remove chicken from broth with a slotted spoon and cool slightly. 2. Meanwhile, in a blender or food processor, combine 1/2 cup of the strawberries, the orange juice, salad oil, lemon peel, lemon juice, sugar, chili powder, salt, and black pepper. Cover; blend or process until smooth. Transfer to a small saucepan. Bring just to a boil. Simmer, uncovered, 5 minutes, stirring occasionally. 3. Thinly slice chicken breasts. In a large bowl, toss together salad greens, remaining strawberries, and chicken. 4. To serve, drizzle warm dressing over salad. Sprinkle with walnuts.

Nutrition facts per serving: 287 calories, 31g protein, 12g carbohydrate, 14g fat (2g saturated), 7g fiber

Whole Wheat Pasta with Ricotta and Vegetables

Makes: 4 servings

Ingredients

- 8 ounces dried whole wheat or whole-grain penne pasta
- 2 1/2 cups broccoli florets
- 1 1/2 cups asparagus or green beans cut into 1-inch pieces
- 1 cup light ricotta cheese
- 1/4 cup snipped fresh basil or 1 tablespoon dried basil, crushed
- 4 teaspoons snipped fresh thyme or 1 teaspoon dried thyme, crushed
- 4 teaspoons balsamic vinegar
- 1 tablespoon olive oil
- 1 garlic clove, minced
- 1/2 teaspoon salt
- 1/2 teaspoon freshly ground black pepper
- 2 large ripe tomatoes, seeded and chopped
- 2 tablespoons grated Parmesan or Romano cheese

Directions: 1. Cook pasta according to package directions, omitting any oil or salt. 2. Add broccoli florets and asparagus or green beans during the last 3 minutes of cooking; drain. 3. In a large serving bowl, combine ricotta cheese, basil, thyme, balsamic vinegar, olive oil, garlic salt, and freshly ground pepper. 4. Add cooked pasta and vegetables to ricotta mixture. Add chopped tomatoes. Toss to combine Sprinkle each serving with grated cheese; serve immediately.

Nutrition facts per serving: 361 calories, 16g protein, 55g carbohydrates, 9g fat (2g saturated), 7g fiber

Southwestern Black Bean Cakes with Guacamole

Makes: 4 servings

Ingredients

- 1/2 medium avocado, seeded and peeled
- 1 tablespoon lime juice
- Ground black pepper and salt
- 2 slices whole wheat bread, torn
- 3 tablespoons fresh cilantro leaves
- 2 garlic cloves
- 1 15-ounce can black beans, rinsed and drained
- 1 canned chipotle pepper in adobo sauce
- 1-2 teaspoons adobo sauce
- 1 teaspoon ground cumin
- 1 egg, beaten
- 1 small plum tomato, chopped

Directions: 1. Mash the avocado in a small bowl. Stir in lime juice; season to taste with salt and pepper. Cover and chill until ready to serve2. Place torn bread in a food processor. Cover and process until bread turns into coarse crumbs. Transfer to a large bowl; set aside. 3. Place cilantro and garlic in the food processor. Cover and process until finely chopped. Add the beans, chipotle pepper, adobo sauce, and cumin. Cover and process until beans are coarsely chopped and mixture begins to pull away from the side of the bowl or container.4. Add mixture to bread crumbs. Add egg, combine, and shape into four 1/2-inch-thick patties.5. Lightly grease the rack of a grill pan. Place patties on the rack. Cook over medium-high heat for 8 to 10 minutes, or until patties are heated through, turning once.6. To serve, top patties with guacamole and tomato.

Nutrition facts per serving: 178 calories, 11g protein, 25g carbohydrate, 7g fat (1g saturated), 9g fiber

Thai Chicken-Broccoli Wraps

Makes: 6 servings

Ingredients

- 12 ounces skinless, boneless chicken-breast strips
- 1/4 teaspoon garlic salt
- 1/8 teaspoon black pepper
- Nonstick cooking spray
- 2 cups packaged broccoli slaw
- 1/2 teaspoon ground ginger
- 3 tablespoons creamy peanut butter
- 1 tablespoon reduced-sodium soy sauce
- 1/2 teaspoon minced garlic
- 3 10-inch whole wheat tortillas, warmed

Directions: 1. Sprinkle chicken strips with garlic salt and pepper. Coat a skillet with cooking spray. Add chicken; cook over medium-high heat for 2 to 3 minutes, or until no longer pink. Remove from pan; keep warm. Add broccoli and 1/4 teaspoon of the ground ginger to skillet. Cook and stir for 2 to 3 minutes, or until vegetables are crisp-tender. 2. In a saucepan, combine peanut butter, 2 tablespoons water, soy sauce, minced garlic, and the remaining ginger. Heat over low heat until smooth, whisking constantly. 3. To assemble, spread tortillas with peanut sauce. Top with chicken strips and vegetable mixture. Roll up each tortilla, securing with a toothpick. Cut in half; serve immediately.

Nutrition facts per serving: 191 calories, 18g protein, 16g carbohydrate, 6g fat (1g saturated), 2g fiber

Greek Quinoa and Avocados

Makes: 4 servings

Ingredients

- 1/2 cup uncooked quinoa
- 1 cup water
- 2 Roma (plum) tomatoes, seeded and finely chopped
- 1/2 cup shredded fresh spinach
- 1/3 cup finely chopped red onion
- 2 tablespoons lemon juice
- 2 tablespoons olive oil
- 1/2 teaspoon salt
- Spinach leaves
- 2 avocados, pitted, peeled, and sliced
- 1/3 cup crumbled feta cheese

Directions: 1. Bring quinoa and water to a boil in a small saucepan. Reduce heat; cover and simmer for 15 minutes, or until liquid is absorbed. 2. In a medium bowl, stir together quinoa, tomatoes, spinach, and onion. 3. In a small bowl, whisk together lemon juice, oil, and salt. Mix with quinoa. 4. Place spinach on plates with avocado slices and quinoa. Sprinkle with feta.

Nutrition facts per serving: 332 calories, 7g protein, 27g carbohydrate, 24g fat (5g saturated), 8g fiber

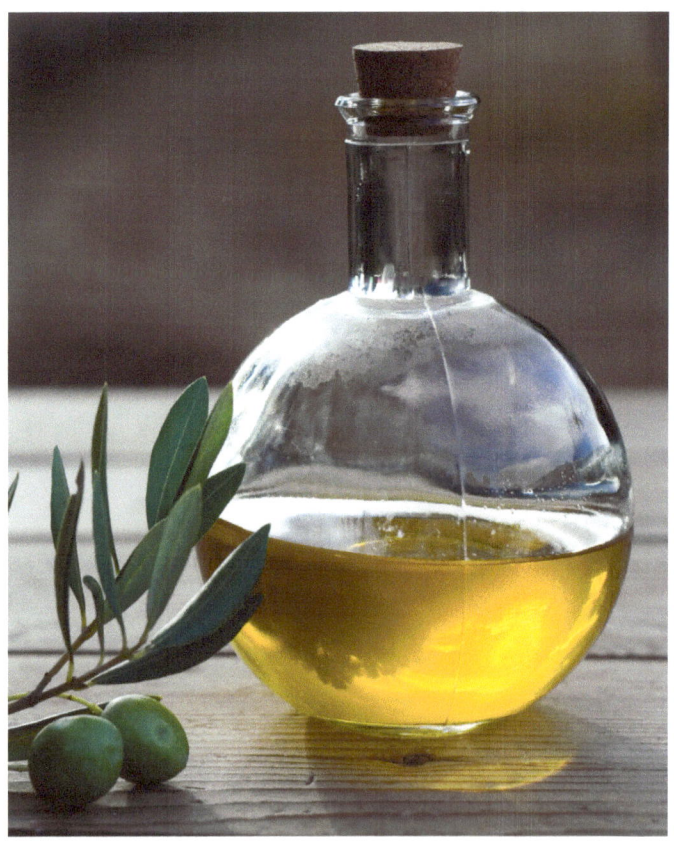

Fat-Burning Snacks

4 whole-grain crackers and 1 ounce reduced-fat cheddar **103 calories**

1 banana dipped in 1/2 ounce melted dark chocolate **176 cal**

Low-fat pudding cup topped with 2/3 cup berries **146 cal**

2 T hummus with 4 baby carrots **66 cal**

10 tortilla chips with 2 tablespoons spicy black bean dip **135 cal**

1/2 cup low-fat ricotta cheese with 1 cup sliced berries and 2 teaspoons honey **209 cal**

1 slice toasted cinnamon raisin bread ,1/2 ounce melted dark chocolate ,1/2 sliced banana **223 cal**

1 c. strawberries blended, 1 tablespoon lime juice ,1 teaspoon honey topped,1 T. coconut **137 cal**

1/3 c.dried apricots dipped in 1/2 ounce melted dark chocolate and 1/4 ounce pistachios **210 cal**

1/2 cup fat-free berry sorbet **120 cal**

2 cups popcorn topped with 1 T. Parmesan cheese **84 cal**

2 hard-boiled eggs with 4 whole-grain crackers **178 cal**

1 flour tortilla topped with 2 chopped slices avocado and 3 T. black beans **197 cal**

1/2 cup blueberries mixed with 1 T. honey and 1/2 cup low-fat plain yogurt **182 cal**

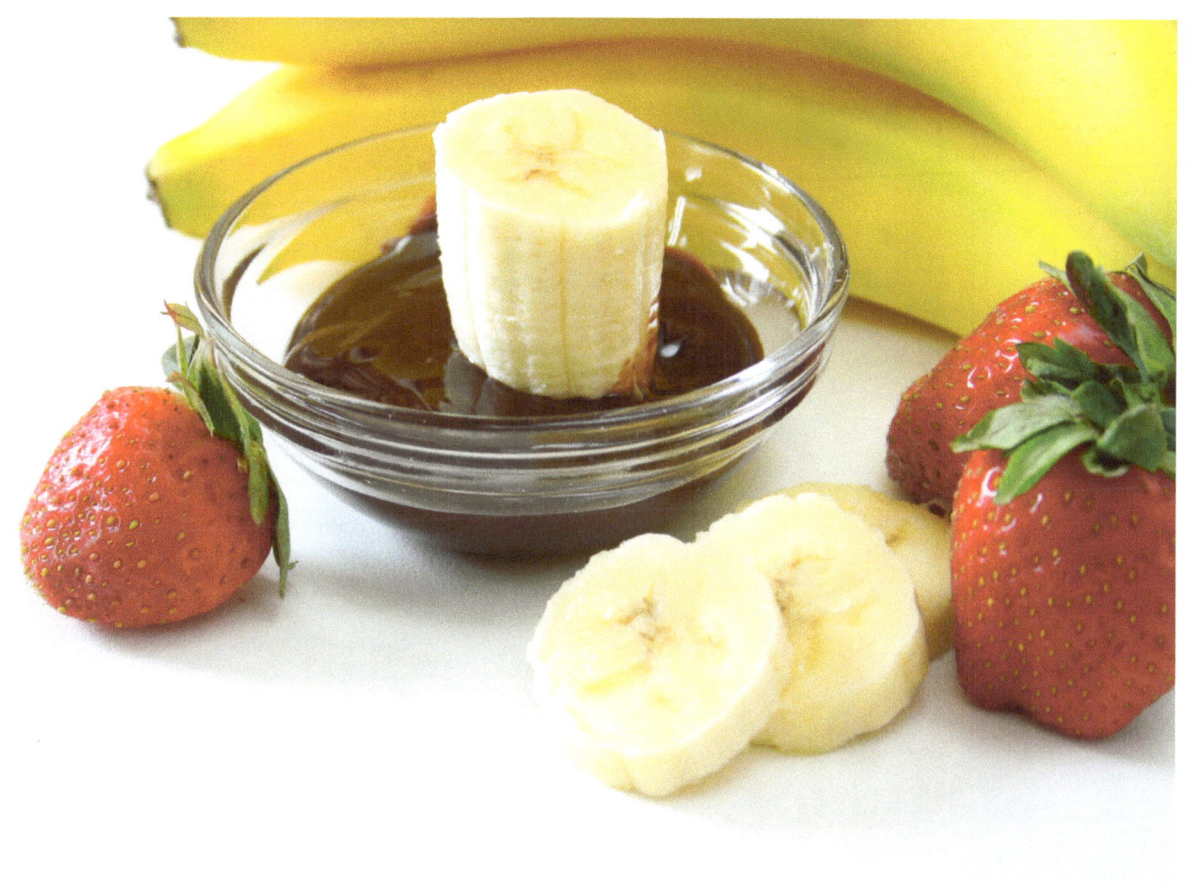

Chapter 5 - Diabetic Diet Menu

The following menu is designed for diabetics who are aiming to lose weight, control blood sugar, and lower cholesterol and triglyceride levels. Adhering to this menu can make a profound difference to your blood glucose and insulin levels. The most import feature of a daily menu is its mix of complexcarbohydrates such as grains, fruits and vegetables, lean proteins and healthy fats. The calorie totals range from 1200-1500 per day.

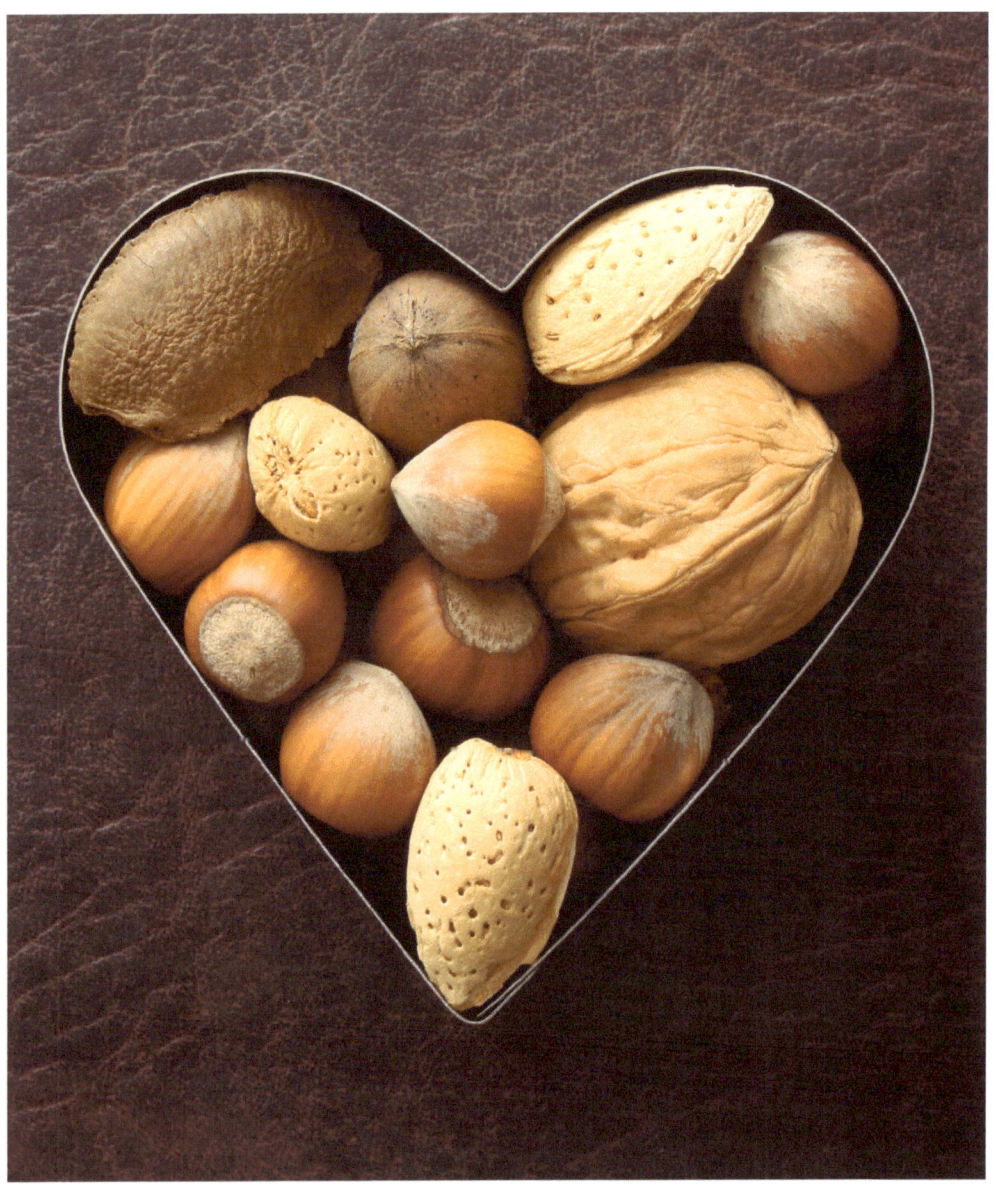

Day 1

Breakfast: 1 small (2 oz.) bran muffin, ½ c. blueberries, 1 c. fat-free milk

Snack: 1 small banana dipped in dark chocolate

Lunch: Spinach salad with 2 tbs. Reduced fat dressing of choice, 1 small whole wheat pita,

2 oz. low-sodium turkey breast, lettuce leaves, tomato slices, 2 tsp. Mustard,

1 orange, 1 c. fat-free milk

Snack: 20 almonds, 6 oz. low-fat yogurt, 1 c. herbal tea or coffee

Dinner: ¼ lb. Raw shrimp, grilled or sauteed in small amount of olive oil, ¾ c. whole wheat pasta

¼ c. black beans, 1 c. steamed broccoli.

Day 2

Breakfast: 2 slices whole-wheat toast, 2 T peanut butter, 1 small banana, 1 c. tea or coffee

Snack: 1 c. green tea, ½ c unsweetened applesauce, 2 T chopped walnuts

Lunch: 2 slices whole wheat bread, 3 oz. lean roast beef, 2 t. mustard, 1 c. cauliflower

Snack: 1 c. fat free milk, 2 small fig cookies

Dinner: 3 oz. chicken breast, sauteed with 1 c. of vegetables of choice, 1 T. olive oil,

2/3 c. brown rice, 1 c. fat free milk

Day 3

Breakfast: ¾ c. bran cereal, 1 c. strawberries, 1 c. fat free milk

Snack: 12 red or green grapes, ½ c. cottage cheese

Lunch: 1 serving beef barley soup (10 oz.), 1 multi grain dinner roll, 1 medium apple

Snack: ¼ c. sunflower seeds, 6 oz. low fat yogurt

Dinner: 6 oz. halibut or other white fish, broiled, 2/3 c. whole wheat couscous, mixed

Green salad with 2 t. reduced fat dressing, 1 c. tea or coffee

Chapter 6 - Gluten Free Meal Ideas

Sample Meal Ideas

Breakfast: eggs, yogurt or cottage cheese, any meat or fish, fruit, nuts, peanut butter

Gluten free toast, rice cakes, smoked salmon

Snacks: corn chips (with salsa or guacomole), nuts, beef jerky (not teriyaki flavor), cheese

Smoothies, kettle chips (naturally gluten free)

L/D: Burrito in a bowl (no tortilla), tacos (in a corn tortilla shell), salads (no croutons or

Blue cheese), lettuce wrapped burger, grilled chicken breast (no bun). Sushi (no soy

Sauce). Any meat, vegetable, fruit, beans, rice, corn, potatoes, fajitas (with corn

Tortillas).

Desserts: Breyers or Haagan Daaz ice cream (it is gluten free) Gluten free cookies, muffins

Chapter 7 - Healthy Substitutions Guide

If your recipe calls for:	Try substituting
All-purpose (plain) flour	Whole-wheat flour
Butter	Applesauce
Creamed soups	Fat-free milk-based soups
Eggs	2 egg whites
Enriched pasta	Whole wheat pasta
Fruit canned in heavy syrup	Fruit canned in its own syrup
Ground beef	chicken or turkey
Table salt	Herbs, spices, fruit juices
White bread	Whole wheat bread
White rice	Brown rice